Eat Your Way to Healthy Skin: The Link between Nutrition and Complexion

Chloe Moreau

Copyright © [2023]

Title: Eat Your Way to Healthy Skin: The Link between Nutrition and Complexion

Author's: Chloe Moreau.

All rights reserved. No part of this publication may be reproduced, stored in a retrieval system, or transmitted in any form or by any means, electronic, mechanical, photocopying, recording, or otherwise, without the prior written permission of the publisher or author, except in the case of brief quotations embodied in critical reviews and certain other non-commercial uses permitted by copyright law.

This book was printed and published by [Publisher's: Chloe Moreau] in [2023]

ISBN:

TABLE OF CONTENTS

Chapter 1: Understanding the Importance of Nutrition for Healthy Skin   06

The Role of Nutrition in Skin Health

Common Skin Problems Associated with Poor Nutrition

The Link between Diet and Complexion

Chapter 2: The Basics of a Skin-Friendly Diet   12

Nutrients Essential for Healthy Skin

Incorporating Antioxidants into Your Diet

Hydration and its Impact on Skin

Chapter 3: Foods to Nourish Your Skin   18

Vitamin-Rich Foods for a Glowing Complexion

Omega-3 Fatty Acids and their Benefits for Skin

The Power of Probiotics for Skin Health

Chapter 4: The Impact of Sugar and Processed Foods on Your Skin   24

Understanding the Effects of Sugar on Skin

Processed Foods and Skin Inflammation

Limiting Harmful Ingredients for Radiant Skin

Chapter 5: The Gut-Skin Connection   30

The Gut Microbiome and its Influence on Skin Health

Healing the Gut for Clearer Skin

Probiotics and Prebiotics for a Healthy Gut and Complexion

Chapter 6: Lifestyle Factors for Healthy Skin   36

The Importance of Sleep for Skin Rejuvenation

Managing Stress for a Clear Complexion

Exercise and its Impact on Skin Health

Chapter 7: Creating a Personalized Skincare Routine   42

Understanding Your Skin Type

Choosing the Right Skincare Products for Your Needs

Incorporating Nutrition into Your Skincare Routine

Chapter 8: Tips for Maintaining Healthy Skin in Different Life Stages — 48

Skin Health during Adolescence and Puberty

Skin Changes during Pregnancy and Menopause

Aging Gracefully: Skin Care in Later Years

Chapter 9: Debunking Common Myths about Nutrition and Skin — 54

Separating Fact from Fiction: The Truth about Chocolate and Acne

Debunking Dieting Myths for Better Skin

Exploring the Impact of Dairy on Complexion

Chapter 10: Embracing a Holistic Approach to Skin Health — 60

Balancing Nutrition, Skincare, and Self-Care

Mindfulness and its Positive Effects on Skin

Achieving Long-Term Skin Health through Sustainable Changes

Conclusion: Transforming Your Complexion through Nutritional Choices — 66

Chapter 1: Understanding the Importance of Nutrition for Healthy Skin

The Role of Nutrition in Skin Health

Proper nutrition plays a vital role in maintaining healthy skin. Our skin is not only the largest organ in our body but also a reflection of our overall health. It is essential to understand that what we eat directly impacts our skin's appearance and complexion. In this subchapter, we will delve into the link between nutrition and skin health, shedding light on how bad nutrition affects a person's appearance.

When we indulge in a diet primarily consisting of processed foods, sugary snacks, and unhealthy fats, it takes a toll on our skin. Such poor nutritional choices can lead to various skin issues, including acne breakouts, dull complexion, and premature aging. Let's explore each of these effects in detail.

Firstly, acne breakouts are often a result of imbalanced nutrition. Foods high in refined sugars and unhealthy fats can trigger inflammation in the body, leading to increased sebum production and clogged pores. Moreover, a lack of essential nutrients like zinc and vitamin A can compromise the skin's ability to heal and regenerate, exacerbating acne-related problems.

Secondly, a diet lacking in vital nutrients can contribute to a dull complexion. Our skin requires a wide array of vitamins, minerals, and antioxidants to maintain its natural radiance. For instance, vitamin C is crucial for collagen production, which gives the skin its firmness and elasticity. A deficiency in this vitamin can result in dull and sagging skin. Similarly, inadequate intake of omega-3 fatty acids, found in fatty fish and walnuts, can lead to dry and lackluster skin.

Lastly, bad nutrition can accelerate the aging process, causing premature wrinkles, fine lines, and sagging skin. Antioxidants, present in fruits and vegetables, protect the skin from free radicals, which are harmful molecules that damage collagen and elastin fibers. By consuming a diet rich in antioxidants, we can slow down the aging process and maintain a youthful appearance. On the other hand, a diet high in processed foods and fried snacks promotes inflammation and oxidative stress, accelerating the formation of wrinkles and contributing to premature aging.

In conclusion, our dietary choices have a profound impact on our skin health and appearance. By nourishing our bodies with a well-balanced diet, rich in fruits, vegetables, whole grains, lean proteins, and healthy fats, we can promote clear, radiant, and youthful-looking skin. It is crucial to prioritize nutrition for the sake of our skin and overall well-being.

Common Skin Problems Associated with Poor Nutrition

Proper nutrition is not only essential for overall health but also plays a significant role in maintaining healthy skin. Our skin is the body's largest organ, and it requires a balanced diet to function optimally. Unfortunately, poor nutrition can have detrimental effects on our skin, leading to various skin problems that can affect our appearance and self-esteem.

One of the most common skin problems associated with poor nutrition is acne. While many factors contribute to acne development, studies have shown that a diet high in refined carbohydrates, sugars, and unhealthy fats can worsen acne symptoms. These foods can spike insulin levels, leading to increased sebum production and inflammation, both of which are key factors in the development of acne. By adopting a more balanced diet rich in fruits, vegetables, whole grains, and lean proteins, individuals can help reduce acne breakouts and achieve clearer skin.

Another skin problem linked to poor nutrition is dryness and flakiness. Inadequate intake of essential fatty acids, such as omega-3 and omega-6, can result in a weakened skin barrier, leading to dry and dehydrated skin. Additionally, insufficient intake of vitamins A, C, and E, which are crucial for skin health, can further exacerbate dryness. To combat this issue, individuals should incorporate foods rich in healthy fats, such as avocados, nuts, and fatty fish, as well as fruits and vegetables high in vitamins into their diet.

Furthermore, poor nutrition can also contribute to premature aging of the skin. A diet lacking in antioxidants, such as vitamins C and E, can leave the skin vulnerable to oxidative stress and damage from free radicals. This can lead to the development of wrinkles, fine lines, and age spots. By consuming a diet abundant in antioxidants through fresh fruits, vegetables, and whole grains, individuals can help protect their skin from premature aging and maintain a youthful complexion.

In conclusion, poor nutrition can have a significant impact on our skin's health and appearance. Acne, dryness, and premature aging are just a few of the common skin problems associated with a lack of proper nutrition. By adopting a balanced diet that includes a variety of fruits, vegetables, whole grains, lean proteins, and healthy fats, individuals can improve their skin's health and achieve a radiant complexion. Remember, what you eat is not only fuel for your body but also nourishment for your skin.

The Link between Diet and Complexion

We have all heard the saying, "You are what you eat." But did you know that what you eat can also affect the appearance of your skin? That's right, the food you put into your body has a direct impact on the health and complexion of your skin. In this subchapter, we will explore the link between diet and complexion and how bad nutrition can affect a person's appearance.

When it comes to maintaining healthy skin, the importance of a well-balanced diet cannot be overstated. Your skin is the largest organ in your body, and it requires essential nutrients to function properly. Without these nutrients, your skin can become dry, dull, and prone to various skin conditions.

One of the key nutrients for healthy skin is antioxidants. Antioxidants help protect your skin from damage caused by free radicals, which can speed up the aging process and lead to wrinkles and fine lines. You can find antioxidants in foods such as berries, dark leafy greens, and nuts. Incorporating these foods into your diet can help promote a youthful complexion.

On the other hand, a diet high in processed foods, sugar, and unhealthy fats can have a detrimental effect on your skin. These types of foods can cause inflammation in the body, which can manifest as acne, redness, and other skin problems. Additionally, sugary foods can lead to glycation, a process that damages collagen and elastin, resulting in sagging and wrinkled skin.

Furthermore, dehydration can also contribute to poor complexion. When you don't drink enough water, your skin becomes dehydrated, leading to dryness and a lackluster appearance. Staying hydrated by consuming plenty of water and eating water-rich foods like cucumbers and watermelon can help keep your skin plump and radiant.

To improve your complexion and achieve healthy skin, it is crucial to make conscious choices about what you eat. A diet rich in fruits, vegetables, lean proteins, and whole grains can provide your skin with the necessary nutrients to thrive. Avoiding processed foods, sugary treats, and excessive alcohol consumption can also do wonders for your complexion.

In conclusion, the link between diet and complexion is undeniable. Your skin reflects what you put into your body, and bad nutrition can have a significant impact on your appearance. By making mindful choices and embracing a healthy, balanced diet, you can nourish your skin from within and achieve a radiant, youthful complexion. Remember, eating your way to healthy skin is not only beneficial for your appearance but also for your overall well-being.

Chapter 2: The Basics of a Skin-Friendly Diet

Nutrients Essential for Healthy Skin

When it comes to achieving healthy and glowing skin, the role of proper nutrition cannot be overstated. Our skin is the largest organ in our body and acts as a protective barrier against external factors. However, it also reflects what is happening inside our body, making it crucial to nourish it from within. In this subchapter, we will explore the key nutrients that are essential for maintaining healthy skin and how their absence can negatively impact our appearance.

One of the most important nutrients for healthy skin is vitamin C. This powerful antioxidant plays a crucial role in the production of collagen, a protein that gives our skin its elasticity and firmness. Without sufficient vitamin C, our skin can become dull, dry, and prone to wrinkles. Citrus fruits, strawberries, bell peppers, and leafy greens are excellent sources of vitamin C that should be included in our daily diet.

Another essential nutrient is vitamin E, which works hand in hand with vitamin C to protect our skin from damage caused by free radicals. Found in nuts, seeds, and vegetable oils, vitamin E helps to moisturize and rejuvenate our skin, keeping it supple and youthful. Deficiencies in this vitamin can lead to dryness, premature aging, and even the formation of scars.

Omega-3 fatty acids are another key nutrient that promotes healthy skin. These healthy fats help to maintain the skin's natural oil barrier, preventing dryness and inflammation. They also support the production of collagen and elastin, resulting in plumper and more resilient skin. Fatty fish like salmon and mackerel, as well as flaxseeds and walnuts, are excellent sources of omega-3 fatty acids that we should incorporate into our diet.

Lastly, the mineral zinc is vital for healthy skin as it supports the function of enzymes involved in collagen synthesis and wound healing. Zinc also helps to regulate oil production, reduce inflammation, and fight acne-causing bacteria. Oysters, lean meats, legumes, and whole grains are all rich sources of zinc that can contribute to clearer and more radiant skin.

In conclusion, maintaining a diet rich in essential nutrients is crucial for healthy skin. Vitamin C, vitamin E, omega-3 fatty acids, and zinc are just a few examples of the nutrients that play vital roles in promoting a radiant complexion. By incorporating these nutrients into our diet, we can nourish our skin from within and enjoy the benefits of a youthful and glowing appearance.

Incorporating Antioxidants into Your Diet

Antioxidants are like superheroes for your skin. They are powerful compounds that protect your cells from damage caused by harmful molecules called free radicals. By neutralizing these free radicals, antioxidants help to reduce inflammation, improve skin elasticity, and promote a healthy complexion. In this subchapter, we will explore the importance of incorporating antioxidants into your diet for healthier, more radiant skin.

First and foremost, it is essential to understand how bad nutrition affects a person's appearance. When you consume a diet high in processed foods, sugary treats, and unhealthy fats, your body becomes overloaded with toxins and lacks the necessary nutrients for optimal skin health. This can lead to a dull complexion, acne breakouts, premature aging, and other skin concerns. However, by making conscious choices to include antioxidant-rich foods in your diet, you can reverse these effects and achieve a glowing complexion.

One of the best ways to introduce antioxidants into your daily meals is by incorporating a variety of colorful fruits and vegetables. These plant-based foods are packed with vitamins, minerals, and phytochemicals that act as antioxidants. Berries, such as blueberries, strawberries, and raspberries, are particularly high in antioxidants like vitamin C and anthocyanins. Citrus fruits like oranges and grapefruits are also excellent sources of vitamin C, which helps to boost collagen production and protect against sun damage.

Leafy greens like spinach, kale, and Swiss chard are loaded with antioxidants like vitamins A and E, as well as lutein and zeaxanthin, which protect against oxidative stress. Additionally, cruciferous vegetables like broccoli, cauliflower, and Brussels sprouts contain sulforaphane, a potent antioxidant that helps to detoxify the skin and reduce inflammation.

Incorporating antioxidant-rich foods into your diet doesn't mean you have to sacrifice taste or variety. Try adding a handful of berries to your morning smoothie, topping your salads with a variety of colorful vegetables, or snacking on antioxidant-rich nuts like almonds and walnuts. You can also experiment with herbs and spices like turmeric, cinnamon, and oregano, which are all rich in antioxidants.

By consciously incorporating antioxidants into your diet, you can nourish your skin from within and enhance your overall appearance. Remember, healthy skin starts from the inside out. So, make it a point to include a rainbow of antioxidant-rich foods in your meals and watch your complexion transform into a radiant, healthy glow.

Hydration and its Impact on Skin

In our quest for healthy, glowing skin, we often overlook one simple yet crucial aspect of skincare – hydration. The importance of staying properly hydrated goes far beyond quenching one's thirst. Adequate hydration plays a pivotal role in maintaining the health and appearance of our skin. This subchapter aims to shed light on the direct relationship between hydration and skin health, revealing the impact dehydration can have on our complexion.

Our skin, the body's largest organ, acts as a protective barrier against external aggressors. It is made up of cells that require water to function optimally. When we neglect to consume enough water, our skin becomes dehydrated, leading to a range of issues like dryness, flakiness, and a dull complexion.

Dehydration affects every skin type, from oily to dry. Contrary to popular belief, dehydration is not a problem exclusive to those with naturally dry skin. Even oily skin can suffer from dehydration, as the oil glands attempt to compensate for the lack of moisture by producing more oil. This can result in an unwanted shiny appearance and an increased risk of breakouts.

Not only does dehydration affect the superficial appearance of the skin, but it also impacts its overall health. When our skin lacks moisture, it becomes more susceptible to damage, fine lines, and wrinkles. Additionally, dehydration can impair the skin's ability to heal itself, leading to a slower recovery from skin conditions such as acne or eczema.

To maintain optimal hydration levels and promote healthy, vibrant skin, it is crucial to prioritize adequate water intake. Experts recommend drinking at least eight glasses of water per day, but individual needs may vary depending on factors such as climate, physical activity, and overall health. Furthermore, incorporating hydrating foods into our diet can provide an additional boost to our skin's moisture levels. Foods rich in water content, such as cucumbers, watermelon, and leafy greens, can help hydrate the skin from within.

In conclusion, hydration is an integral part of any skincare regimen. By ensuring we consume enough water and incorporate hydrating foods into our diet, we can support our skin's natural functions and achieve a healthy, radiant complexion. Remember, the key to healthy skin lies not only in the products we apply externally but also in the nourishment we provide from the inside out.

Chapter 3: Foods to Nourish Your Skin

Vitamin-Rich Foods for a Glowing Complexion

A healthy and radiant complexion is something we all desire, but did you know that what you eat plays a crucial role in achieving that glowing skin? Your skin is the largest organ of your body, and it reflects your overall health and well-being. Poor nutrition can have a significant impact on your appearance, leading to skin problems such as acne, dullness, dryness, and premature aging. However, by incorporating vitamin-rich foods into your diet, you can nourish your skin from within and achieve that enviable glow.

1. Vitamin C: This powerful antioxidant is essential for collagen production, which gives your skin its elasticity and firmness. Citrus fruits like oranges, grapefruits, and lemons are excellent sources of vitamin C. Additionally, berries, kiwis, and bell peppers are also packed with this vital nutrient.

2. Vitamin E: Known for its ability to protect the skin from oxidative damage, vitamin E is found in foods like almonds, sunflower seeds, spinach, and avocados. Including these foods in your diet will help promote healthy skin cell turnover, leaving you with a youthful and glowing complexion.

3. Vitamin A: Crucial for maintaining healthy skin cells and preventing dryness, vitamin A can be found in sweet potatoes, carrots, spinach, and kale. These foods contain beta-carotene, which is converted into vitamin A in the body, ensuring a smooth and supple complexion.

4. Omega-3 Fatty Acids: These healthy fats are essential for maintaining the integrity of your skin cell membranes and reducing inflammation. Fatty fish like salmon, mackerel, and sardines are excellent sources of omega-3 fatty acids. Alternatively, you can opt for plant-based sources such as flaxseeds, chia seeds, and walnuts.

5. Zinc: This mineral plays a crucial role in regulating oil production and reducing inflammation, making it beneficial for acne-prone skin. Foods rich in zinc include oysters, lean meats, pumpkin seeds, and lentils.

By incorporating these vitamin-rich foods into your diet, you can improve your skin's health and achieve a glowing complexion. Remember, it's not just about what you put on your skin but also what you put into your body that matters. So, start nourishing your skin from within and watch as your complexion transforms into a radiant and healthy glow.

Omega-3 Fatty Acids and their Benefits for Skin

When it comes to achieving healthy and glowing skin, the importance of good nutrition cannot be emphasized enough. Our skin is a reflection of our overall health, and what we eat plays a crucial role in maintaining its vitality. One group of nutrients that has gained significant attention for its skin benefits is omega-3 fatty acids.

Omega-3 fatty acids are a type of polyunsaturated fat that is found in certain foods, such as fatty fish (salmon, sardines, and mackerel), walnuts, flaxseeds, and chia seeds. These essential fats are not produced by our bodies, so it's important to incorporate them into our diet.

One of the primary benefits of omega-3 fatty acids for the skin is their anti-inflammatory properties. Inflammation is often the root cause of various skin issues, including acne, eczema, and psoriasis. By including omega-3 fatty acids in our diet, we can help reduce inflammation and improve the overall appearance of our skin.

Omega-3 fatty acids also play a crucial role in maintaining the skin's moisture barrier. This barrier is responsible for keeping our skin hydrated and protecting it from external factors such as pollution and harsh weather conditions. When our skin's moisture barrier is compromised, it can lead to dryness, irritation, and premature aging. By consuming foods rich in omega-3 fatty acids, we can support the integrity of our skin's barrier and promote optimal hydration.

Furthermore, omega-3 fatty acids have been shown to enhance collagen production, a protein that is essential for maintaining the structure and elasticity of our skin. As we age, our natural collagen levels decline, leading to the formation of wrinkles and sagging skin. By incorporating omega-3 fatty acids into our diet, we can support collagen synthesis and slow down the aging process, resulting in a more youthful complexion.

In addition to these direct benefits for the skin, omega-3 fatty acids also contribute to overall health and well-being. They have been shown to reduce the risk of heart disease, lower blood pressure, and improve brain function. By nourishing our bodies with these essential fats, we can achieve not only healthy skin but also a healthier and happier life.

To reap the benefits of omega-3 fatty acids for your skin, aim to include fatty fish, nuts, and seeds in your diet regularly. Consider adding flaxseed or chia seeds to your morning smoothie or enjoy a delicious salmon dinner once or twice a week. By making these simple dietary changes, you can harness the power of omega-3 fatty acids and unlock the path to radiant and healthy skin.

Remember, good nutrition is the foundation for a beautiful complexion. By embracing the power of omega-3 fatty acids, you can eat your way to healthy skin and enjoy the numerous benefits it brings to your overall well-being.

The Power of Probiotics for Skin Health

In our quest for healthy and radiant skin, we often overlook the importance of maintaining a healthy gut. Surprisingly, the key to achieving a flawless complexion lies within our digestive system. Probiotics, often referred to as the "good bacteria," have gained significant attention in recent years for their remarkable benefits not only on our gut health but also on our skin.

Probiotics are live microorganisms that, when consumed in adequate amounts, confer health benefits to the host. They play a crucial role in balancing the bacteria in our gut, promoting better digestion and absorption of nutrients. However, their benefits extend far beyond our gut, making them a powerful ally for achieving optimal skin health.

When our gut is overloaded with harmful bacteria, it can lead to various skin issues such as acne, eczema, and rosacea. By introducing probiotics into our diet, we can restore the balance of bacteria in our gut, leading to a healthier complexion. Probiotics help strengthen the skin's natural barrier, reducing inflammation and improving overall skin function.

One of the key mechanisms through which probiotics benefit the skin is by supporting the immune system. A healthy gut flora strengthens our immune response, helping to combat harmful bacteria and pathogens that can trigger skin conditions. Additionally, probiotics have been found to increase the production of ceramides, essential lipids that maintain the skin's moisture and prevent dryness and wrinkles.

Probiotics also have a significant impact on the overall appearance of our skin. They enhance collagen production, a protein responsible for skin elasticity and firmness. By maintaining adequate levels of collagen, probiotics can help reduce the signs of aging, such as fine lines and wrinkles, giving us a more youthful complexion.

To harness the power of probiotics for skin health, it's essential to incorporate probiotic-rich foods into our diet. Fermented foods like yogurt, kefir, sauerkraut, and kimchi are excellent sources of probiotics. Alternatively, probiotic supplements can be taken to ensure an adequate intake of beneficial bacteria.

In conclusion, the power of probiotics for skin health cannot be underestimated. By maintaining a healthy gut flora, we can improve our skin's appearance, reduce inflammation, and combat various skin conditions. So, next time you're looking to enhance your skincare routine, remember to nourish your gut with probiotic-rich foods or supplements. Your skin will thank you for it!

Chapter 4: The Impact of Sugar and Processed Foods on Your Skin

Understanding the Effects of Sugar on Skin

In our modern society, sugar has become a ubiquitous ingredient in our diets. From sweet treats to beverages, it seems almost impossible to avoid its tempting allure. However, what many people fail to realize is that excessive sugar consumption can have detrimental effects on our skin. In this subchapter, we will delve into the topic of understanding the effects of sugar on our skin, shedding light on the connection between nutrition and complexion.

Sugar, in its various forms, has the ability to wreak havoc on our skin. When consumed in excess, it can trigger a process known as glycation, which damages collagen and elastin fibers in our skin. These fibers are responsible for maintaining its firmness and elasticity, leading to premature signs of aging such as wrinkles, fine lines, and sagging skin. Furthermore, glycation also results in the production of harmful molecules called advanced glycation end products (AGEs), which contribute to inflammation and oxidative stress, further exacerbating skin damage.

Not only does sugar accelerate the aging process, but it can also lead to the development of skin conditions such as acne. High sugar intake increases insulin levels, which in turn triggers the release of hormones called androgens. These hormones stimulate the production of sebum, an oily substance that clogs pores and creates a breeding ground for acne-causing bacteria. Additionally, sugar consumption can disrupt the balance of gut bacteria, leading to inflammation and a weakened immune system, both of which play a role in the development of acne.

To maintain a healthy complexion, it is essential to reduce our sugar intake and opt for more nutritious alternatives. Incorporating a diet rich in fruits, vegetables, lean proteins, and whole grains can provide the necessary nutrients for healthy skin. Antioxidant-rich foods such as berries, leafy greens, and nuts help combat oxidative stress and inflammation caused by sugar. Moreover, staying hydrated by drinking plenty of water helps flush out toxins and keeps the skin hydrated and supple.

In conclusion, understanding the effects of sugar on our skin is crucial for maintaining a healthy complexion. By recognizing the connection between nutrition and our appearance, we can make informed choices about our dietary habits and take proactive steps towards improving our skin's health. With a mindful approach to nutrition, we can truly eat our way to healthy skin.

Processed Foods and Skin Inflammation

In today's fast-paced world, it is all too easy to rely on convenience foods and processed snacks to fuel our bodies. However, what many people fail to realize is that these processed foods can have a detrimental effect on our skin. In this subchapter, we will explore the link between processed foods and skin inflammation and how bad nutrition can negatively impact a person's appearance.

Processed foods are typically high in added sugars, unhealthy fats, and artificial ingredients. These ingredients can wreak havoc on our skin by disrupting the delicate balance of our body's natural systems. One of the major consequences of consuming too many processed foods is the development of skin inflammation.

Skin inflammation occurs when our bodies react to foreign substances or irritants. When we consume processed foods, our bodies often perceive them as harmful substances, triggering an inflammatory response. This response can manifest itself in various ways, including acne breakouts, redness, and even more severe conditions such as eczema or psoriasis.

The high sugar content in processed foods is particularly problematic for our skin. When we consume excess sugar, it causes a spike in our blood sugar levels, leading to a process called glycation. Glycation damages collagen and elastin, two essential proteins responsible for keeping our skin firm and youthful. Consequently, the breakdown of collagen and elastin leads to premature aging, fine lines, and wrinkles.

Furthermore, processed foods are often lacking in essential nutrients and antioxidants that are crucial for maintaining healthy skin. These foods are typically stripped of their natural vitamins and minerals during processing, leaving us with empty calories and little nutritional value. Without the necessary nutrients, our skin's ability to repair itself and fight off free radicals is compromised, resulting in a dull and lackluster complexion.

To improve the health of our skin, it is essential to reduce our consumption of processed foods and opt for whole, unprocessed foods instead. Incorporating a diet rich in fruits, vegetables, lean proteins, and whole grains can provide our bodies with the necessary nutrients to promote skin health and reduce inflammation.

In conclusion, the link between processed foods and skin inflammation is undeniable. By understanding the negative effects of bad nutrition on our appearance, we can make more informed choices about the foods we consume. By prioritizing whole, unprocessed foods, we can nourish our bodies from the inside out, leading to healthier, more radiant skin.

Limiting Harmful Ingredients for Radiant Skin

In today's fast-paced world, we are constantly bombarded with advertisements for skincare products promising flawless, radiant skin. However, what many people fail to realize is that achieving healthy, glowing skin starts from within. Our diet plays a crucial role in determining the appearance of our skin, and consuming harmful ingredients can have detrimental effects on our complexion.

How Bad Nutrition Affects a Person's Appearance

The saying, "you are what you eat," couldn't be more accurate when it comes to the health of our skin. Poor nutrition can lead to a range of skin issues, including acne, dryness, and premature aging. When we consume foods high in sugar, processed oils, and artificial additives, our skin becomes more prone to inflammation and breakouts.

One ingredient that wreaks havoc on our skin is sugar. Excessive sugar consumption can lead to a process called glycation, where sugar molecules attach to proteins in our body, including collagen and elastin, causing them to become stiff and less resilient. This results in sagging skin and the formation of wrinkles.

Another harmful ingredient is processed oils, such as trans fats and hydrogenated oils. These oils can cause inflammation in the body, leading to acne breakouts and a dull complexion. Additionally, they can disrupt the balance of essential fatty acids in our skin, resulting in dryness and flakiness.

Artificial additives, commonly found in processed foods and drinks, can also take a toll on our skin. These additives, including artificial sweeteners and food colorings, can trigger allergic reactions and inflammation in the body. This can manifest as redness, rashes, and even eczema.

To achieve radiant skin, it is crucial to limit the consumption of these harmful ingredients. Instead, focus on incorporating whole, nutrient-dense foods into your diet. Fresh fruits and vegetables, lean proteins, and healthy fats, such as avocados and nuts, are all excellent choices for promoting healthy skin.

Additionally, staying hydrated is key for maintaining a youthful complexion. Make sure to drink plenty of water throughout the day to keep your skin hydrated and plump.

In conclusion, the food we consume plays a significant role in the appearance of our skin. By limiting harmful ingredients such as sugar, processed oils, and artificial additives, and instead opting for nutrient-rich foods, we can achieve radiant, healthy skin. Remember, true beauty starts from within, and nourishing our bodies with the right ingredients will reflect on our complexion.

Chapter 5: The Gut-Skin Connection

The Gut Microbiome and its Influence on Skin Health

When it comes to achieving healthy, radiant skin, most people tend to focus on external factors such as skincare products and treatments. However, the secret to a glowing complexion may actually lie within our gut. The gut microbiome, composed of trillions of bacteria and other microorganisms residing in our digestive system, plays a crucial role in maintaining overall health, including the health of our skin.

The gut microbiome not only helps with digestion and nutrient absorption but also plays a vital role in modulating our immune system and regulating inflammation throughout the body. When the balance of bacteria in our gut is disrupted, it can lead to various health issues, including skin problems. This is due to the connection between the gut and the skin known as the gut-skin axis.

Research has shown that an imbalanced gut microbiome can contribute to skin conditions such as acne, eczema, and even premature aging. When harmful bacteria outnumber the beneficial ones, it can trigger an inflammatory response, leading to the release of inflammatory molecules that can manifest on the skin as redness, irritation, and blemishes.

Moreover, a compromised gut can impair the body's ability to eliminate toxins efficiently. This can result in a buildup of toxins, which may further contribute to skin problems. On the other hand, a healthy and diverse gut microbiome promotes proper digestion, enhances nutrient absorption, and helps eliminate toxins effectively, ultimately leading to clearer and healthier skin.

So, how can we nurture our gut microbiome and support our skin health? The answer lies in our diet. Consuming a nutrient-rich, balanced diet that includes plenty of fiber, fruits, vegetables, and fermented foods can help promote a diverse and thriving gut microbiome. Fermented foods, such as yogurt, sauerkraut, and kefir, are particularly beneficial as they contain live bacteria that can help replenish and diversify the gut microbiome.

Additionally, it is crucial to avoid or limit processed foods, refined sugars, and unhealthy fats, as they can negatively impact the gut microbiome and contribute to skin problems. Drinking plenty of water and staying hydrated is also essential for maintaining skin health, as it helps flush out toxins and keeps the skin hydrated from within.

In conclusion, the gut microbiome plays a significant role in influencing our skin health. By nourishing our gut with a balanced, nutritious diet and avoiding harmful food choices, we can promote a diverse and thriving gut microbiome, leading to clearer, healthier, and more radiant skin. Remember, true beauty starts from within!

Healing the Gut for Clearer Skin

The Link between Nutrition and Complexion

Have you ever wondered why your skin doesn't seem to glow as it should, no matter how many skincare products you try? The answer might lie within your gut. Surprisingly, the state of your gut health plays a crucial role in the appearance of your skin. In this subchapter, we will explore the fascinating connection between gut health and clearer skin. By understanding this relationship, you can take steps to heal your gut and achieve the radiant complexion you've always desired.

Our modern diets, filled with processed foods, refined sugars, and artificial additives, can wreak havoc on our gut health. When our gut becomes imbalanced, it can lead to inflammation, poor nutrient absorption, and a weakened immune system. These issues can manifest as various skin conditions, such as acne, eczema, and even premature aging.

When the gut is unhealthy, it becomes permeable, allowing toxins and harmful bacteria to enter the bloodstream. This triggers an immune response, leading to inflammation that can manifest on the skin's surface. By healing the gut, we can reduce inflammation and promote the body's natural ability to repair and rejuvenate our skin.

So, how can we heal our gut and achieve clearer skin? It all starts with the foods we eat. A diet rich in whole, unprocessed foods is essential for gut health. Incorporating plenty of fruits and vegetables, lean proteins, and healthy fats can provide the necessary nutrients for optimal skin health.

In addition to a nutrient-dense diet, certain foods have been shown to specifically promote gut healing. Fermented foods like sauerkraut, kimchi, and kefir contain probiotics that help restore the balance of beneficial bacteria in the gut. These bacteria play a crucial role in maintaining a healthy gut environment.

Furthermore, incorporating foods high in fiber, such as whole grains, legumes, and vegetables, can support a healthy gut by promoting regular bowel movements and aiding in the removal of toxins from the body.

In conclusion, healing the gut is vital for achieving clearer skin. By adopting a nutritious diet and incorporating gut-healing foods, you can support your body's natural ability to repair and rejuvenate your skin. Remember, what you put into your body is just as important as what you put on your skin. So, take charge of your gut health and unlock the secret to a radiant complexion.

Probiotics and Prebiotics for a Healthy Gut and Complexion

Maintaining a healthy gut is not only crucial for our overall well-being but also plays a significant role in the appearance of our skin. The food we consume has a direct impact on our gut health, which in turn affects our complexion. In this subchapter, we will explore the importance of probiotics and prebiotics in promoting a healthy gut and achieving a radiant complexion.

Probiotics, often referred to as "good bacteria," are live microorganisms that offer numerous health benefits when consumed. They help restore the natural balance of bacteria in our gut, improving digestion and nutrient absorption. A healthy gut flora is vital for a properly functioning immune system, which can help combat skin conditions such as acne and eczema. Including probiotics in our diet can also reduce inflammation and promote a more youthful and vibrant complexion.

Foods rich in probiotics include yogurt, kefir, sauerkraut, kimchi, and kombucha. Adding these to our meals or enjoying them as snacks can help replenish the beneficial bacteria in our gut and promote a healthy complexion. Additionally, probiotic supplements are available for those who may have difficulty incorporating enough probiotic-rich foods into their diet.

Prebiotics, on the other hand, are non-digestible fibers that serve as food for the probiotics in our gut. They help nourish the beneficial bacteria, allowing them to thrive and multiply. By consuming prebiotics, we can support the growth of good bacteria, which in turn helps maintain a healthy gut and radiant skin.

Some examples of prebiotic-rich foods include garlic, onions, bananas, asparagus, and oats. Incorporating these foods into our meals can provide us with the necessary nutrients to support a healthy gut flora and improve our complexion.

When considering the link between nutrition and complexion, it is essential to focus on the health of our gut. By including probiotics and prebiotics in our diet, we can create an optimal environment for beneficial bacteria to flourish, leading to improved digestion, better absorption of nutrients, and a more radiant complexion.

In conclusion, probiotics and prebiotics play a crucial role in promoting a healthy gut, which is directly linked to the appearance of our skin. By incorporating probiotic-rich foods and consuming prebiotics, we can support the growth of beneficial bacteria in our gut, leading to improved digestion and a more radiant complexion. So, let's prioritize our gut health and nourish it with the right foods to achieve healthy, glowing skin.

Chapter 6: Lifestyle Factors for Healthy Skin

The Importance of Sleep for Skin Rejuvenation

When it comes to achieving healthy and glowing skin, many people focus solely on their skincare routine and diet. While these factors play a significant role in maintaining good skin, one crucial aspect that often gets overlooked is sleep. Adequate sleep is essential for skin rejuvenation and overall health. In this subchapter, we will explore the importance of sleep in achieving healthy and radiant skin.

Sleep is often referred to as the body's "reset" button. During sleep, our bodies repair and regenerate cells, including the skin cells. Lack of sleep can lead to a host of skin problems, including dullness, uneven tone, and premature aging. When we are sleep-deprived, our bodies produce more stress hormones, such as cortisol, which can cause inflammation and break down collagen, leading to wrinkles and sagging skin.

Additionally, during deep sleep, our bodies release growth hormones that aid in the repair and renewal of skin cells. These growth hormones help to maintain the skin's elasticity and firmness, giving it a youthful appearance. Without enough sleep, this natural rejuvenation process is disrupted, resulting in a tired and lackluster complexion.

Moreover, sleep deprivation can affect the balance of moisture in the skin. When we sleep, our bodies regulate hydration levels, preventing dryness and promoting a healthy moisture barrier. Without adequate sleep, the skin's ability to retain moisture is compromised, leading to dry and flaky skin.

Furthermore, lack of sleep can contribute to the formation of dark circles and under-eye bags. When we don't get enough rest, blood vessels expand, causing the skin under our eyes to appear darker. Moreover, fluid can accumulate in the area, resulting in puffy and swollen eyes. These visible signs of fatigue can make us look older and less vibrant.

To ensure optimal skin rejuvenation, it is crucial to prioritize getting enough sleep. Aim for seven to nine hours of quality sleep every night. Establish a bedtime routine that promotes relaxation, such as turning off electronic devices an hour before bed, practicing mindfulness or meditation, and creating a comfortable sleep environment.

In conclusion, sleep is not just a luxury; it is a vital component of achieving healthy and radiant skin. By understanding the importance of sleep for skin rejuvenation, we can make the necessary changes in our lifestyle to prioritize restful sleep. Incorporating sufficient sleep into our daily routine, along with a healthy diet and skincare regimen, will help us achieve the complexion we desire and maintain overall well-being.

Managing Stress for a Clear Complexion

Stress is an inevitable part of life, and it can have a profound impact on our overall well-being, including our complexion. In this subchapter, we will explore how stress affects our skin and provide practical tips on managing stress for a clear complexion.

It is well-known that stress can trigger various skin issues, such as acne breakouts, eczema flare-ups, or even premature aging. When we experience stress, our body releases cortisol, a hormone that can disrupt the balance of other hormones in our body. This hormonal imbalance can lead to increased oil production, clogged pores, and inflammation, resulting in unwanted skin conditions.

To manage stress effectively and maintain a clear complexion, it is crucial to adopt healthy coping mechanisms. One of the most effective ways to reduce stress is through regular exercise. Engaging in physical activities like jogging, yoga, or swimming helps release endorphins, also known as "feel-good" hormones, which can reduce stress levels and promote a healthy complexion.

Another important aspect of stress management is getting enough sleep. Lack of sleep can worsen stress and increase the risk of skin problems. Aim for seven to eight hours of quality sleep each night to allow your body and mind to recharge. Creating a relaxing bedtime routine, such as reading a book or taking a warm bath, can help you unwind and improve the quality of your sleep.

In addition to exercise and sleep, incorporating stress-reducing activities into your daily routine can work wonders for your complexion. Consider practicing mindfulness or meditation, which can help calm your mind and reduce stress levels. Deep breathing exercises or engaging in hobbies that you enjoy, such as painting, gardening, or playing a musical instrument, can also provide a much-needed break from the demands of daily life.

Furthermore, it is essential to nourish your body with a balanced diet to support your skin's health during stressful times. Avoid consuming excessive amounts of sugary foods, caffeine, and processed snacks, as they can exacerbate stress levels and negatively impact your complexion. Instead, focus on eating nutrient-rich foods, such as fruits, vegetables, lean proteins, and whole grains, which provide essential vitamins and minerals for healthy skin.

Managing stress for a clear complexion requires a holistic approach that addresses both the mind and body. By adopting healthy coping mechanisms, engaging in stress-reducing activities, and nourishing your body with a balanced diet, you can minimize the impact of stress on your skin and improve your overall well-being. Remember, self-care is not selfish but rather an essential step towards achieving healthy, glowing skin.

Exercise and its Impact on Skin Health

Regular exercise not only contributes to overall physical fitness but also plays a significant role in maintaining healthy and glowing skin. When it comes to skin health, most people focus solely on skincare products and treatments, neglecting the importance of incorporating exercise into their routine. In this subchapter, we will explore how exercise can positively impact the health and appearance of your skin.

Exercise promotes healthy blood circulation, which is crucial for delivering oxygen and nutrients to the skin cells. When you engage in physical activity, your heart rate increases, and blood vessels dilate, allowing for enhanced blood flow to the skin. This increased circulation helps nourish the skin cells, resulting in a radiant and youthful complexion.

Additionally, exercise aids in the detoxification process by encouraging perspiration. Sweating is the body's natural way of eliminating toxins, dirt, and impurities from the skin. Regular exercise not only opens up your pores but also helps flush out harmful substances that can clog them, leading to acne breakouts and dull skin.

Moreover, exercise has been shown to reduce stress levels, which can have a profound impact on your skin's health. Stress is known to trigger various skin conditions, such as acne, eczema, and psoriasis. By engaging in physical activity, you release endorphins, which are natural mood boosters that help alleviate stress. Consequently, this reduction in stress levels can improve the overall appearance of your skin, promoting a clear and vibrant complexion.

Furthermore, exercise promotes collagen production, a vital protein responsible for maintaining the skin's elasticity and firmness. As we age, collagen production naturally declines, leading to sagging skin and wrinkles. However, regular exercise stimulates collagen synthesis, helping to minimize the signs of aging and promoting a more youthful appearance.

In conclusion, exercise is not only beneficial for your physical well-being but also for the health of your skin. By incorporating regular exercise into your routine, you can improve blood circulation, aid in detoxification, reduce stress levels, and promote collagen production. These factors contribute to a healthier complexion, allowing you to achieve the clear, radiant skin you desire. So, lace up those sneakers, hit the gym, or engage in any physical activity of your choice, and watch your skin reap the rewards of your efforts.

Chapter 7: Creating a Personalized Skincare Routine

Understanding Your Skin Type

Your skin is a remarkable organ that protects your body from external factors such as pollution, harmful UV rays, and bacteria. It also plays a crucial role in regulating body temperature and eliminating toxins. However, not everyone's skin is the same. Each person has a unique skin type, which can significantly impact their overall appearance and health. In this subchapter, we will delve into the different skin types and how understanding yours can help you achieve healthy and glowing skin.

There are four main skin types: oily, dry, combination, and normal. Oily skin tends to produce excess sebum, making it prone to acne and a shiny appearance. On the other hand, dry skin lacks moisture and often feels tight or flaky. Combination skin is a mix of both oily and dry, with the T-zone (forehead, nose, and chin) being oily while the cheeks and other areas are dry. Lastly, normal skin is well-balanced and has a healthy glow.

Understanding your skin type is vital because it allows you to choose the right skincare products and adopt a suitable diet. Bad nutrition can have a detrimental impact on your skin, regardless of your skin type. Consuming a diet high in processed foods, sugary snacks, and unhealthy fats can lead to inflammation, breakouts, and premature aging. On the other hand, a diet rich in antioxidants, vitamins, and minerals can promote healthy skin by reducing inflammation, boosting collagen production, and improving overall complexion.

For those with oily skin, incorporating foods high in omega-3 fatty acids, such as fatty fish, flaxseeds, and walnuts, can help regulate sebum production and reduce acne. Dry skin types can benefit from consuming foods rich in healthy fats, like avocados, olive oil, and nuts, to improve skin hydration and elasticity. Combination skin types should focus on a balanced diet that includes a variety of fruits, vegetables, whole grains, and lean proteins to maintain skin health in both oily and dry areas. Lastly, individuals with normal skin can maintain their healthy complexion by eating a well-rounded diet and staying hydrated.

By understanding your skin type and the impact of nutrition on your complexion, you can make informed choices about what you eat and how you care for your skin. Remember, healthy skin starts from within, and a nourishing diet can significantly contribute to your overall appearance. So, let's embark on this journey together and eat our way to healthy, glowing skin!

Choosing the Right Skincare Products for Your Needs

When it comes to achieving healthy and radiant skin, it's not just about what you eat, but also about the skincare products you use. The market is flooded with countless options, making it overwhelming to find the right products for your specific skin concerns. However, with a little knowledge and understanding, you can choose skincare products that will help you achieve the complexion you desire.

Firstly, it's important to identify your skin type. Is your skin oily, dry, combination, or sensitive? Knowing your skin type will help you select products that cater to its unique needs. For example, if you have oily skin, look for oil-free or mattifying products that control shine and prevent breakouts. On the other hand, if your skin is dry, opt for moisturizing and hydrating products that restore moisture and prevent flakiness.

Once you have determined your skin type, consider your specific skincare concerns. Are you struggling with acne, fine lines, dark spots, or dullness? Different ingredients target different concerns, so it's essential to look for products that address your specific issues. For acne-prone skin, products containing salicylic acid or benzoyl peroxide can be beneficial. If you're concerned about signs of aging, look for products with ingredients like retinol, hyaluronic acid, or peptides.

Another factor to consider is the quality and reputation of the brand. Look for skincare brands that have a good track record and use high-quality ingredients. Read customer reviews and seek recommendations from trusted sources to ensure that the products you choose are effective and safe.

Furthermore, it's crucial to understand that skincare is not a one-size-fits-all approach. What works for someone else may not work for you. Therefore, it's important to experiment and be patient when trying out new products. Give each product enough time to see if it produces the desired results before moving on to the next one.

Lastly, don't forget about the importance of a good skincare routine. Choosing the right products is just the first step; using them consistently and correctly will make all the difference. Cleanse, tone, moisturize, and protect your skin from the sun's harmful rays with sunscreen. Consistency and dedication to a skincare routine will help you achieve and maintain healthy, glowing skin.

In conclusion, choosing the right skincare products for your needs is essential for achieving healthy and radiant skin. Identify your skin type, consider your specific concerns, and choose products that cater to those needs. Research brands, read reviews, and be patient in finding what works best for you. Combine this with a consistent skincare routine, and you'll be on your way to achieving the complexion you've always desired.

Incorporating Nutrition into Your Skincare Routine

Your skin is a reflection of your overall health and well-being. It is the largest organ in your body and acts as a protective barrier against harmful external factors. While many people focus solely on external skincare products to achieve healthy skin, the secret to a radiant complexion lies in incorporating nutrition into your skincare routine.

The link between nutrition and complexion is undeniable. What you eat plays a significant role in the health and appearance of your skin. Poor nutrition can lead to a range of skin issues, including acne, dullness, dryness, and premature aging. By understanding how bad nutrition affects your appearance, you can take steps to improve your diet and achieve healthy, glowing skin.

One of the key ways bad nutrition affects your skin is through inflammation. Consuming excessive amounts of processed foods, sugary treats, and unhealthy fats can trigger inflammation in the body, resulting in redness, irritation, and breakouts. Incorporating a diet rich in antioxidants, such as fruits, vegetables, and whole grains, can help combat this inflammation and promote clearer skin.

Another way bad nutrition impacts your appearance is by depriving your skin of essential nutrients. Nutrient deficiencies can lead to a lackluster complexion, dryness, and increased susceptibility to environmental damage. To counteract this, focus on consuming a variety of vitamins and minerals that are beneficial for skin health, such as vitamin C, vitamin E, zinc, and omega-3 fatty acids. These can be found in foods like citrus fruits, nuts, seeds, fish, and leafy greens.

Moreover, a diet high in refined carbohydrates and sugar can accelerate the aging process by causing the breakdown of collagen and elastin, two proteins that keep your skin firm and supple. To promote youthful skin, opt for complex carbohydrates like whole grains and reduce your intake of sugary foods and drinks.

Incorporating nutrition into your skincare routine doesn't stop at what you eat. You can also nourish your skin from the outside by using skincare products that contain natural, nutrient-rich ingredients. Look for products with antioxidants like green tea extract, vitamin C, and coenzyme Q10, as they can protect your skin from free radicals and promote a more youthful complexion.

In conclusion, bad nutrition can have a detrimental effect on your appearance, causing skin issues and premature aging. By incorporating nutrition into your skincare routine, both internally and externally, you can improve the health and vitality of your skin. Remember to eat a balanced diet, rich in antioxidants and essential nutrients, and choose skincare products that nourish and protect your skin. By embracing this holistic approach to skincare, you can eat your way to healthy, radiant skin.

Chapter 8: Tips for Maintaining Healthy Skin in Different Life Stages

Skin Health during Adolescence and Puberty

During adolescence and puberty, the body goes through various changes, and one area that is greatly affected is the skin. The teenage years can be a challenging time for many individuals, as they may experience acne breakouts, oily skin, and other skin-related issues. This subchapter aims to shed light on the importance of maintaining proper nutrition during this crucial period of growth and development.

One of the primary reasons why adolescents and teenagers suffer from skin problems is due to bad nutrition. The food we consume plays a vital role in the overall health of our skin. A poor diet lacking in essential nutrients can lead to an imbalance in hormones, which often results in skin issues such as acne.

Processed foods, sugary snacks, and fast food are commonly consumed by teenagers due to their convenience and taste. However, these foods are usually high in refined sugars, unhealthy fats, and artificial additives, all of which can wreak havoc on the skin. Excessive consumption of these foods can cause inflammation, clog pores, and increase sebum production, leading to acne breakouts.

To maintain healthy skin during adolescence and puberty, it is crucial to focus on a balanced diet rich in fruits, vegetables, lean proteins, and whole grains. These foods contain essential vitamins, minerals, and antioxidants that promote skin health. Vitamins A, C, and E are particularly beneficial for skin health, as they help repair damaged skin cells, fight free radicals, and reduce inflammation.

Furthermore, staying hydrated is essential for maintaining healthy skin. Water helps flush out toxins from the body and keeps the skin hydrated and supple. Adolescents should aim to drink at least eight glasses of water per day to support optimal skin health.

In addition to proper nutrition, it is essential to establish a good skincare routine during adolescence. Cleansing the skin twice a day, using a gentle cleanser and moisturizer suitable for their skin type, can help keep the skin clean and prevent breakouts.

Overall, paying attention to nutrition and adopting a healthy lifestyle during adolescence and puberty can significantly improve skin health. By making conscious choices about the foods we consume and taking care of our skin, we can achieve a clear and glowing complexion during this crucial stage of life.

Skin Changes during Pregnancy and Menopause

Pregnancy and menopause are two significant phases in a woman's life that bring about various physical and hormonal changes. These changes often manifest on the skin, presenting different challenges and concerns. Understanding these skin changes is crucial for maintaining healthy and glowing skin throughout these transformative periods.

During pregnancy, hormonal fluctuations play a vital role in skin changes. Many women experience an increase in oil production, leading to acne breakouts. This is primarily due to elevated levels of androgens, a group of hormones responsible for stimulating oil glands. Additionally, increased blood flow during pregnancy can result in a rosy complexion, commonly referred to as the "pregnancy glow." However, some women also encounter pigmentation issues such as melasma or "mask of pregnancy," which causes dark patches on the face.

Another common skin concern during pregnancy is stretch marks. As the body rapidly expands to accommodate the growing baby, the skin's elasticity is put to the test, often resulting in stretch marks on the abdomen, thighs, breasts, and buttocks. While stretch marks cannot be completely prevented, keeping the skin well-hydrated and maintaining a healthy weight can help minimize their appearance.

Menopause, on the other hand, brings its own set of skin challenges. As estrogen levels decline, the skin becomes thinner, drier, and more vulnerable to damage. Wrinkles and fine lines become more apparent, and skin may appear dull and lackluster. Additionally, decreased collagen production leads to a loss of elasticity, contributing to sagging and drooping skin.

Hot flashes, a common symptom of menopause, can also impact the skin. The sudden rise in body temperature causes blood vessels to dilate, resulting in flushed and red skin. Some women may experience increased sensitivity and irritation as well.

While these skin changes during pregnancy and menopause may seem daunting, there are ways to support the skin's health and mitigate their effects. Proper nutrition plays a crucial role in maintaining healthy skin throughout these phases. A balanced diet rich in antioxidants, vitamins, and minerals can help nourish the skin from within, combat oxidative stress, and promote a youthful complexion.

Incorporating foods like fruits, vegetables, whole grains, lean proteins, and healthy fats can provide essential nutrients for skin health. Hydration is also key, as it helps maintain skin elasticity and aids in the natural detoxification process.

By understanding and addressing the skin changes that occur during pregnancy and menopause, individuals can make informed choices to support their skin's health. With the right nutrition and skincare routine, it is possible to navigate these transformative phases while maintaining a radiant and healthy complexion.

Aging Gracefully: Skin Care in Later Years

As we age, our bodies undergo numerous changes, including those that affect our skin. The natural aging process combined with external factors such as sun exposure, pollution, and poor nutrition can lead to the development of wrinkles, age spots, and a dull complexion. However, by adopting a proper skin care routine and making healthy dietary choices, we can slow down the signs of aging and promote a radiant complexion in our later years.

The link between nutrition and complexion is a crucial aspect of maintaining healthy skin throughout our lives. Poor nutrition can have a detrimental effect on our appearance, leading to dryness, inflammation, and premature aging. When we consume a diet high in processed foods, sugary treats, and unhealthy fats, our skin suffers. These foods lack essential nutrients that support skin health, such as vitamins, minerals, and antioxidants.

To counteract the negative impact of bad nutrition on our appearance, it is important to prioritize a diet rich in fruits, vegetables, whole grains, and lean proteins. These foods are packed with vitamins A, C, and E, which are vital for skin health. Vitamin A helps to repair and maintain skin tissues, vitamin C promotes collagen production, and vitamin E protects against oxidative damage. Additionally, antioxidants found in colorful fruits and vegetables help to neutralize harmful free radicals, preventing premature aging.

In addition to a healthy diet, establishing a comprehensive skin care routine is crucial for aging gracefully. Regularly cleansing, exfoliating, and moisturizing the skin helps to remove impurities, stimulate cell turnover, and maintain hydration. It is also important to incorporate sunscreen into our daily routine, as the harmful UV rays from the sun are one of the primary causes of skin aging.

Furthermore, adopting lifestyle habits that promote overall wellness can also contribute to healthy skin in later years. Engaging in regular exercise, managing stress levels, and getting sufficient sleep all play a role in maintaining a youthful complexion. Exercise improves circulation, aiding in the delivery of nutrients to the skin, while stress reduction techniques and quality sleep promote skin cell regeneration.

In conclusion, taking care of our skin as we age is essential for maintaining a youthful and radiant complexion. By understanding the link between nutrition and skin health and making conscious choices to prioritize a nutrient-rich diet, establish a comprehensive skin care routine, and adopt a healthy lifestyle, we can age gracefully and enjoy healthy skin well into our later years. Remember, it is never too late to start taking care of your skin – the results will be well worth the effort.

Chapter 9: Debunking Common Myths about Nutrition and Skin

Separating Fact from Fiction: The Truth about Chocolate and Acne

One of the most common misconceptions when it comes to bad nutrition and its effects on our appearance is the belief that chocolate causes acne. For years, chocolate has been unfairly blamed for those pesky pimples that seem to pop up at the most inconvenient times. But is there any truth to this claim, or is it just another myth?

The truth is, there is no scientific evidence to support the idea that chocolate directly causes acne. Acne is a complex skin condition that is influenced by a variety of factors, such as genetics, hormones, and overall skin health. While diet can play a role in the development of acne, it is not solely responsible for its occurrence.

So why has chocolate been singled out as a culprit? One reason could be the confusion between correlation and causation. Many people who suffer from acne also happen to enjoy eating chocolate. This association has led to the assumption that chocolate must be the cause, when in reality, it may just be a coincidence.

In fact, recent studies have shown that the link between chocolate and acne is weak, if not entirely nonexistent. A review published in the Journal of Clinical and Aesthetic Dermatology concluded that there is no significant evidence to support the idea that chocolate consumption directly leads to acne formation. Other factors, such as high glycemic index foods and dairy products, have been found to have a stronger association with acne development.

That being said, it is important to note that not all chocolate is created equal. Dark chocolate, in particular, contains antioxidants and flavonols that can actually benefit the skin. These compounds have been shown to improve blood flow, protect against sun damage, and reduce inflammation. So, while chocolate may not directly cause acne, choosing high-quality dark chocolate in moderation can be a healthier option for your overall skin health.

In conclusion, separating fact from fiction is crucial when it comes to understanding the relationship between chocolate and acne. While chocolate alone is unlikely to be the sole cause of acne, it is important to maintain a balanced diet and consider other factors that may contribute to skin issues. By focusing on overall nutrition and skin health, we can make informed choices that promote a clear and healthy complexion.

Debunking Dieting Myths for Better Skin

In our quest for healthy, glowing skin, we often turn to various diets and fads that promise quick results. However, many of these dieting myths can actually do more harm than good when it comes to our complexion. In this chapter, we will debunk some of the most common dieting myths and shed light on how bad nutrition affects a person's appearance.

Myth #1: Cutting out all fats leads to better skin. One of the most prevalent myths is that all fats are bad for our skin. In reality, our bodies need healthy fats to maintain supple skin. Omega-3 fatty acids, found in foods like salmon, avocados, and walnuts, are essential for reducing inflammation and maintaining skin elasticity. So, instead of eliminating fats altogether, focus on incorporating the right kinds of fats into your diet.

Myth #2: A crash diet will give you flawless skin. Crash diets, which involve severe calorie restriction, may help you lose weight quickly, but they wreak havoc on your skin. When you drastically reduce your calorie intake, your body lacks essential nutrients, leading to dull, dry, and sallow-looking skin. Opt for a balanced diet that includes a variety of fruits, vegetables, whole grains, lean proteins, and healthy fats to nourish your skin from within.

Myth #3: Cutting out carbs is the key to clear skin. Carbohydrates have been unfairly demonized in recent years, with many people believing that they are the culprit behind skin issues like acne. While excessive consumption of refined carbohydrates can contribute to skin problems, eliminating carbs altogether is not the solution. Complex carbohydrates, such as whole grains, provide essential vitamins and minerals that promote healthy skin. Instead of avoiding carbs, focus on choosing high-quality, unprocessed options.

Myth #4: Drinking lots of water guarantees hydrated skin. While staying hydrated is crucial for overall health, drinking copious amounts of water alone won't automatically give you plump, hydrated skin. Hydration also comes from consuming foods rich in water content, like fruits and vegetables. Additionally, factors like genetics, climate, and skincare routine play a significant role in skin hydration. So, ensure you're not solely relying on water intake, but also incorporate hydrating foods and moisturizers into your daily routine.

In conclusion, it's important to debunk these dieting myths to understand how bad nutrition can affect our skin. Instead of falling for quick fixes and restrictive diets, focus on nourishing your body with a well-balanced diet that includes a variety of nutrients. By providing your skin with the right nutrition, you will not only achieve a healthier complexion but also experience overall well-being.

Exploring the Impact of Dairy on Complexion

When it comes to achieving healthy and glowing skin, we often focus on skincare products and treatments without realizing the significant role that nutrition plays in our complexion. In this subchapter, we delve into the impact of dairy on our skin and how it can affect our overall complexion.

Dairy products such as milk, cheese, and yogurt have long been considered staples in many people's diets. However, recent research has shown that dairy consumption may have a profound impact on our skin health. Many individuals experience skin issues such as acne, eczema, and rosacea, and it's essential to understand how our dietary choices can contribute to these conditions.

One of the main culprits in dairy that affects our complexion is hormones. Dairy cows are often given synthetic hormones to increase milk production, and these hormones can transfer to the milk and other dairy products we consume. These hormones, such as insulin-like growth factor 1 (IGF-1), can stimulate oil production in our skin, leading to clogged pores and breakouts.

Furthermore, dairy products contain lactose, a type of sugar that may trigger inflammation in the body. Inflammation is a key factor in various skin conditions, including acne and eczema. By reducing or eliminating dairy from your diet, you may experience a decrease in inflammation and an improvement in your complexion.

Another reason why dairy can negatively impact our skin is due to its high glycemic index. Consuming high-glycemic foods can cause a spike in blood sugar levels, leading to increased insulin production.

This can result in excess sebum production, inflammation, and ultimately, acne breakouts.

It's important to note that everyone's body is unique, and while dairy may have a negative impact on one person's complexion, it may not affect another person in the same way. To determine if dairy is contributing to your skin issues, consider eliminating it from your diet for a few weeks and observing any changes in your complexion.

Remember, a healthy and radiant complexion starts from within. By paying attention to the impact of dairy on our skin, we can make informed dietary choices to support our skin health. Experimenting with alternative sources of calcium and nutrients, such as leafy greens, nuts, and seeds, can provide us with the necessary nutrients for healthy skin without the potential negative effects of dairy.

In conclusion, exploring the impact of dairy on our complexion is crucial for understanding how our dietary choices can affect our skin health. By being aware of the potential negative effects of dairy, we can make informed decisions about our diet to maintain a healthy and glowing complexion.

Chapter 10: Embracing a Holistic Approach to Skin Health

Balancing Nutrition, Skincare, and Self-Care

In today's fast-paced world, it is easy to overlook the importance of maintaining a healthy lifestyle, especially when it comes to nutrition and skincare. We often prioritize our hectic schedules over taking care of ourselves, which can have a detrimental effect on our overall appearance. In this subchapter, we will explore the link between nutrition and complexion, shedding light on how bad nutrition can significantly impact a person's appearance.

When it comes to our skin, what we put into our bodies is just as important as what we put on our skin. A poor diet lacking in essential nutrients can lead to a dull complexion, acne, premature aging, and various other skin issues. Consuming excessive amounts of processed foods, sugary drinks, and unhealthy fats can lead to inflammation, which can manifest as redness, puffiness, and even skin conditions like eczema or psoriasis.

Moreover, a deficiency in vital nutrients such as vitamins A, C, E, and omega-3 fatty acids can weaken the skin's protective barrier, making it more prone to damage from environmental factors like pollution and UV rays. This can result in dryness, sensitivity, and an increased risk of developing wrinkles and fine lines.

To combat these negative effects, it is crucial to adopt a balanced and nutritious diet. Incorporating foods rich in antioxidants, such as berries, leafy greens, and nuts, can help fight oxidative stress and promote a healthy complexion. Additionally, including foods high in collagen-building nutrients like vitamin C (found in citrus fruits and bell peppers) and omega-3 fatty acids (found in fatty fish and flaxseeds) can enhance skin elasticity and reduce the appearance of wrinkles.

While nutrition plays a vital role in maintaining healthy skin, it is equally important to establish a skincare routine that complements your diet. Regularly cleansing, exfoliating, and moisturizing your skin can help remove impurities, unclog pores, and keep your complexion vibrant. It is also essential to choose skincare products that are free from harsh chemicals and are suitable for your skin type.

Finally, self-care should not be overlooked in the pursuit of healthy skin. Stress, lack of sleep, and poor lifestyle choices can contribute to skin issues and an unhealthy appearance. Taking time for relaxation, getting enough sleep, and managing stress through activities like yoga or meditation can greatly improve your complexion.

In conclusion, balancing nutrition, skincare, and self-care is essential for maintaining healthy skin and a vibrant appearance. By adopting a wholesome diet, following a consistent skincare routine, and prioritizing self-care, you can achieve a radiant complexion that reflects your overall well-being. Remember, investing in your health and taking care of yourself is not just a luxury but a necessity for long-term beauty and vitality.

Mindfulness and its Positive Effects on Skin

In today's fast-paced world, it's easy to get caught up in the hustle and bustle of life, often neglecting our own well-being. One aspect of our health that is often overlooked is the condition of our skin. Many of us spend countless hours and dollars on skincare products, hoping to achieve that elusive glow. However, what if I told you that the key to healthy skin lies not only in what you put on your skin but also in your state of mind?

Mindfulness, the practice of being fully present in the moment, has been gaining popularity in recent years for its numerous health benefits. It's not just about sitting cross-legged and meditating; it's about cultivating a sense of awareness and appreciation for the present moment in all aspects of your life, including your skincare routine.

When it comes to the appearance of our skin, stress plays a significant role. High levels of stress can lead to a variety of skin problems, including acne, eczema, and premature aging. By practicing mindfulness, we can reduce stress levels, leading to healthier skin.

One of the ways mindfulness positively affects our skin is by reducing inflammation. Stress triggers the release of cortisol, a hormone that can cause inflammation in the body. By practicing mindfulness and managing stress levels, we can lower cortisol production, resulting in calmer skin and reduced redness.

Furthermore, mindfulness can improve our overall skincare routine. By being present and fully engaged in the process, we can choose products that are suitable for our skin type and address specific concerns effectively. Additionally, being mindful while applying skincare products allows us to massage our face gently, improving blood circulation and promoting a healthy, radiant complexion.

Moreover, mindfulness can enhance the effectiveness of our skincare products. By being in the present moment, we can fully absorb the benefits of the products we use. Instead of mindlessly going through the motions, take a few extra seconds to appreciate the texture, scent, and overall experience of applying each product. This simple act of mindfulness can enhance the efficacy of the products and ultimately improve your skin's health.

In conclusion, mindfulness has a profound impact on our overall well-being, including the condition of our skin. By practicing mindfulness, we can reduce stress levels, manage inflammation, and enhance the effectiveness of our skincare routine. So, the next time you embark on your skincare journey, take a moment to be present, appreciate the process, and enjoy the positive effects it has on your skin.

Achieving Long-Term Skin Health through Sustainable Changes

When it comes to achieving healthy, glowing skin, most people focus solely on topical treatments and skincare products. However, what many fail to realize is that true skin health starts from within. Your diet plays a crucial role in determining the condition of your skin, and making sustainable changes to your nutrition can lead to long-term skin health.

We all know that consuming a diet high in processed foods, sugary drinks, and unhealthy fats can negatively impact our overall health. But did you know that bad nutrition can also affect your appearance, particularly your skin? Skin conditions such as acne, eczema, and premature aging can often be linked to a poor diet.

The main culprit behind these skin issues is inflammation. When you consume a diet high in processed foods and sugary treats, it can trigger an inflammatory response in the body, leading to various skin problems. On the other hand, a diet rich in whole foods, fruits, vegetables, and healthy fats can help reduce inflammation and promote skin health.

To achieve long-term skin health, it is essential to make sustainable changes to your diet and lifestyle. Start by incorporating more fruits and vegetables into your meals. These nutrient-packed foods are rich in antioxidants, vitamins, and minerals that can nourish your skin from the inside out. Aim for a variety of colors to ensure you're getting a wide range of nutrients.

Additionally, focus on consuming healthy fats such as avocados, nuts, and fatty fish. These fats are essential for maintaining the integrity of your skin barrier, keeping it hydrated and protected. Avoiding processed foods, sugary drinks, and excessive alcohol can also do wonders for your skin's appearance.

Remember, achieving long-term skin health is a journey, and it requires consistency and commitment. It may take time to see noticeable changes, but by making sustainable changes to your diet and lifestyle, you'll be on the right path towards healthier, more radiant skin.

In conclusion, bad nutrition can have a significant impact on your skin's appearance. By adopting a diet rich in whole foods, fruits, vegetables, and healthy fats, you can reduce inflammation and promote long-term skin health. Remember, you are what you eat, and your skin reflects your inner health. So, start making sustainable changes today and eat your way to healthy skin!

Conclusion: Transforming Your Complexion through Nutritional Choices

In this book, "Eat Your Way to Healthy Skin: The Link between Nutrition and Complexion," we have explored the profound impact that our nutritional choices can have on our skin. We have delved into the ways in which bad nutrition can negatively affect a person's appearance, and the steps we can take to transform our complexion through better dietary habits.

Our skin is the largest organ in our body, and it reflects our overall health and well-being. When we neglect our nutrition, we deprive our skin of the essential nutrients it needs to thrive. This can result in a variety of skin issues, including acne, dryness, dullness, and premature aging. By understanding the link between nutrition and complexion, we can make informed choices to improve the health and appearance of our skin.

One of the most significant ways in which bad nutrition affects our appearance is through inflammation. Consuming a diet high in processed foods, sugar, and unhealthy fats can trigger an inflammatory response in our body. This inflammation can manifest on our skin as redness, puffiness, and acne breakouts. On the other hand, incorporating anti-inflammatory foods such as fruits, vegetables, whole grains, and omega-3 fatty acids can help reduce inflammation and promote a more radiant complexion.

Another crucial aspect of nutrition that impacts our skin is hydration. Dehydration can lead to dry, flaky skin, and make fine lines and wrinkles more apparent. Drinking an adequate amount of water throughout the day is essential for maintaining skin hydration. Additionally, incorporating hydrating foods such as cucumbers, watermelon, and leafy greens can further support skin hydration.

Furthermore, the role of antioxidants in our diet cannot be overstated. Antioxidants help neutralize free radicals, which are unstable molecules that can damage our skin cells and contribute to premature aging. By consuming a variety of antioxidant-rich foods like berries, dark leafy greens, and green tea, we can protect our skin from oxidative stress and promote a more youthful complexion.

In conclusion, the choices we make regarding our nutrition have a profound impact on our skin's health and appearance. By understanding how bad nutrition affects our complexion, we can take proactive steps to transform our skin through better dietary habits. Incorporating anti-inflammatory foods, staying hydrated, and consuming antioxidant-rich foods can all contribute to a healthier, more vibrant complexion. Remember, your skin deserves the best nutrition, so make wise choices and watch your complexion transform.

www.ingramcontent.com/pod-product-compliance
Lightning Source LLC
LaVergne TN
LVHW052003060526
838201LV00059B/3817